YOUR GUIDE TO KIDNEY HEALTH

A Practical Guide to Preventing and Managing Kidney Disease

SAMANTHA JOLLY

Table of Contents

Abstract

Your Guide to Kidney Health: A Practical Guide to Preventing and Managing Kidney Disease is a comprehensive resource for anyone who wants to learn more about kidney health and how to prevent and manage kidney disease. The book covers everything from the basics of kidney anatomy and function to the latest information on prevention and treatment. It also includes practical tips on how to make healthy lifestyle choices that can protect your kidneys.

Whether you are at risk for kidney disease or you are already living with the condition, Your Guide to Kidney Health is an essential resource for you.

The book is written by an experienced healthcare professional, with help of a nephrologist, a registered dietitian, and a certified diabetes educator.

The book is based on the latest scientific evidence and guidelines from leading medical organizations.

The book is written in a clear and easy-to-understand style, and it is packed with information that can help you take care of your kidneys and live a healthy life.

Introduction

Your kidneys are two bean-shaped organs that are located in the lower back, just below the rib cage. They are responsible for filtering waste products from the blood and helping to regulate blood pressure, electrolyte balance, and red blood cell production.

Kidney disease is a condition that damages the kidneys and impairs their ability to function properly. There are many different types of kidney disease, but the most common are chronic kidney disease (CKD) and acute kidney injury (AKI).

CKD is a progressive condition that can lead to kidney failure if it is not treated. AKI is a sudden onset of kidney failure that can be caused by a number of factors, such as infection, dehydration, or certain medications.

Kidney disease affects millions of people around the world, and it is a major cause of death and disability. However, kidney disease is often preventable, and there are many things that you can do to protect your kidneys and keep them healthy.

This book

This book is a practical guide to preventing and managing kidney disease. It is written for people who are at risk for kidney disease, people who have been diagnosed with kidney disease, and their caregivers.

The book covers a wide range of topics, including:

- The anatomy and function of the kidneys
- The causes, risk factors, and symptoms of kidney disease
- How to prevent kidney disease
- How to manage kidney disease
- The latest treatments for kidney disease
- Living with kidney disease
- The importance of regular check-ups and screenings

The book is written in a clear and easy-to-understand style, and it is packed with information that can help you take care of your kidneys and live a healthy life.

After reading this book, you will know:

- How the kidneys work and why they are important
- What causes kidney disease and who is at risk
- How to prevent kidney disease
- How to manage kidney disease
- The latest treatments for kidney disease
- What it is like to live with kidney disease
- How to get the support you need

How to use this book

This book is a reference guide, so you can use it as a resource whenever you have questions about kidney disease. You can also use the book to help you create a plan to protect your kidneys and manage your kidney disease.

If you are concerned about your kidney health, or if you have been diagnosed with kidney disease, I encourage you to talk to your doctor. Your doctor can help you assess your risk for kidney disease and develop a plan to protect your kidneys.

I also encourage you to join a support group or find other resources that can help you learn more about kidney disease and how to manage it. There are many resources available, and you can find them by searching online or talking to your doctor.

Taking care of your kidneys is important

Your kidneys are essential organs, and they play a vital role in your health. By taking care of your kidneys, you can help to prevent kidney disease and live a long and healthy life.

I hope you find this book helpful. I have written it with the goal of providing you with the information you need to take care of your kidneys and live a healthy life.

Thank you for reading.

Chapter 1
Introduction to the Kidneys

The kidneys are two bean-shaped organs that are found in the lower back, just below the rib cage. They are responsible for cleaning waste products from the blood and helping to control blood pressure, electrolyte balance, and red blood cell production.

The kidneys are essential organs, and they play a key part in maintaining good health. Kidney disease is a disorder that damages the kidneys and impairs their ability to work properly. There are many different kinds of kidney disease, but the most common are chronic kidney disease (CKD) and acute kidney injury (AKI).

CKD is a progressive disease that can lead to kidney failure if it is not handled. AKI is a rapid start of kidney failure that can be caused by a number of factors, such as infection, dehydration, or certain drugs.

Kidney disease affects millions of people around the world, and it is a big cause of death and disability. However, kidney disease is often prevented, and there are many things that you can do to protect your kidneys and keep them healthy.

What are the kidneys?

The kidneys are two bean-shaped organs that are found in the lower back, just below the rib cage. They are about the size of a hand, and they weigh about 12 ounces each.

The kidneys are made up of millions of tiny cleaning units called nephrons. Each nephron is responsible for removing waste products from the blood and making urine.

The kidneys also make hormones that help to control blood pressure, electrolyte balance, and red blood cell production.

Anatomy of the Kidneys

The kidneys are found in the retroperitoneum, which is the space behind the peritoneum, the lining of the abdominal region. The right kidney is somewhat lower than the left kidney because of the stomach.

The kidneys are covered by a layer of fat that helps to protect them. The kidneys are also linked to the ureters, which are tubes that carry water from the kidneys to the bladder.

What do the kidneys do?

The kidneys have a number of important tasks, including:

- Filtering waste products from the blood: The kidneys filter about 125 milliliters of blood per minute. This blood is passed through the nephrons, where waste products are removed and urine is created.

- Regulating blood pressure: The kidneys create a hormone called renin, which helps to control blood pressure. Renin causes the body to create angiotensin II, which causes blood vessels to constrict and blood pressure to rise.

- Balancing electrolytes: The kidneys help to balance the amounts of ions in the blood, such as sodium, potassium, and calcium. Electrolytes are important for a number of body processes, including muscle contraction, nerve transmission, and fluid balance.

- Producing red blood cells: The kidneys make a hormone called erythropoietin, which prompts the bone marrow to create red blood cells. Red blood cells carry oxygen to the tissues, so it is important to have a good amount of red blood cells.

Kidney Disease

Kidney disease is a disorder that damages the kidneys and impairs their ability to work properly. There are many different kinds of kidney disease, but the most common are chronic kidney disease (CKD) and acute kidney injury (AKI).

What are the different types of kidney disease?

There are many different kinds of kidney disease, but the most common are chronic kidney disease (CKD) and acute kidney injury (AKI).

Chronic kidney disease (CKD)

CKD is a progressive disease that damages the kidneys and affects their ability to work properly. CKD is generally identified when the kidneys have lost more than 20% of their function.

CKD can be caused by a number of causes, including high blood pressure, diabetes, and family background. There is no cure for CKD, but it can be controlled with medicine and lifestyle changes.

Acute kidney damage (AKI)

AKI is a rapid start of kidney failure that can be caused by a number of factors, such as infection, dehydration, or certain drugs. AKI is normally reversible, but it can lead to lasting kidney damage if it is not addressed.

How does kidney disease affect the body

Kidney disease can affect the body in a number of ways, including:

- Waste product buildup: When the kidneys are not working properly, waste products can build up in the blood. This can lead to signs such as tiredness, nausea, and vomiting.

- Fluid imbalance: The kidneys help to control the body's fluid balance. When the kidneys are not working properly, fluid can build up in the body, leading to swelling in the hands, feet, and legs.

- Electrolyte imbalance: The kidneys help to balance the amounts of ions in the blood.

When the kidneys are not working properly, electrolyte changes can occur, leading to signs such as muscle cramps, weakness, and confusion.

- High blood pressure: Kidney problems can cause high blood pressure. High blood pressure can hurt the kidneys further, making kidney disease worse.

- Heart disease: kidney disease can increase the risk of heart disease. People with renal illness often pass away from heart disease.

How to prevent kidney disease

There are a number of things that you can do to avoid kidney disease, including:

- Control your blood pressure: High blood pressure is a big risk factor for kidney disease. Keep your blood pressure under control by eating a healthy diet, moving regularly, and taking medicine if necessary.

- Manage your diabetes: Diabetes is another major risk factor for kidney disease. Work with your doctor to keep your blood sugar levels under control if you have diabetes.

- Get regular checkups: If you are at risk for kidney disease, talk to your doctor about getting regular checkups. Your doctor can check your blood pressure, blood sugar, and kidney health.

- Make good living choices: There are a number of other living choices that you can make to help protect your kidneys, such as:

- Eating a healthy diet: A healthy meal is low in salt, potassium, and protein. It is also necessary to drink enough of fluids, especially water.

- Exercise on a regular basis: Exercise helps to regulate your blood pressure and blood sugar levels. It also helps to keep your weight down, which is important for kidney health.

- Quit smoking: Smoking harms the kidneys and increases the risk of kidney disease.

- Avoid dangerous substances: Avoid using illegal drugs and excessive amounts of drink. These chemicals can hurt the kidneys.

Kidney disease is a dangerous illness, but it is often preventable. By making healthy living choices and getting regular checkups, you can help to protect your kidneys and keep them healthy.

Chapter 2
Risk Factors for Kidney Disease

A dangerous sickness that may affect people of all ages is kidney disease. Your chance of having kidney disease can rise due to a variety of causes, such as:

- High blood pressure: The main risk factor for renal disease is high blood pressure. Kidney failure may result from damage to the blood arteries in the kidneys brought on by high blood pressure.

- Diabetes: Another significant risk factor for kidney disease is diabetes. Diabetes makes the kidneys work harder to filter blood, which might harm them.

- Family history: You are more prone to get kidney disease if there is a history of the ailment in your family.

- Age: Older persons are more likely to have kidney disease.

- Race and ethnicity: Compared to white Americans, those of African descent, Hispanic descent, and Native American descent are more prone to acquire renal disease.

- Nonsteroidal anti-inflammatory drugs (NSAIDs) are among the medicines that might harm the kidneys.

- Acute kidney injury: If left untreated, acute kidney injury (AKI) can develop into chronic kidney disease (CKD).

- Obesity: Obesity increases the chance of developing kidney disease among other illnesses.

- Smoking: Smoking harms the kidneys and raises the possibility of developing renal disease.

- Growing older: As people age, their risk of kidney disease rises.

How to Determine Your Kidney Disease Risk

You may conduct a variety of activities to determine your risk for kidney disease, such as:

- Repetitive checkups: Your doctor can examine your kidney function, blood pressure, and blood sugar levels.

- Inquire about your family history with your doctor: Your doctor can go over your risk with you if kidney disease runs in your family.

- Obtain a kidney disease screening: You can ask your doctor to do a kidney disease screening on you if you are worried about your chance of developing the ailment.

How to Lower Your Chances of Contracting Kidney Disease

You may do a variety of things to lower your risk of kidney disease, such as:

- Maintain a healthy blood pressure: The main risk factor for renal disease is high blood pressure. Maintaining a healthy blood pressure level might assist to safeguard your kidneys.

- Maintain control of your blood sugar levels if you have diabetes by working with your doctor.

- Make healthy lifestyle decisions. You may support your kidneys by making a variety of different lifestyle decisions, such as:

- Having a balanced diet: Protein, potassium, and salt are all low in a balanced diet. A lot of fluids should be consumed, especially water.

- Regular exercise Your blood pressure and blood sugar levels can be managed with exercise. Additionally, it aids in maintaining a healthy weight, which is crucial for kidney function.

- Give up smoking: Smoking harms the kidneys and raises the possibility of developing renal disease.

- Avoid using dangerous substances, such as alcohol in excess and illicit narcotics. The kidneys may be harmed by these chemicals.

Despite being a severe sickness, kidney disease is frequently avoidable. You may contribute to protecting and maintaining the health of your kidneys by leading a healthy lifestyle and seeing the doctor frequently.

Additional Details

A plethora of knowledge regarding kidney illness is available from the National Kidney Foundation (NKF), including information on risk factors, symptoms, and available treatments. The NKF website may be found at https://www.kidney.org/.

Another group that disseminates knowledge regarding kidney illness is the American Society of Nephrology (ASN). The ASN website may be accessed at https://www.asn.org/.

Consult your doctor if you have any concerns regarding the health of your kidneys. Your physician can determine your risk for renal disease and make suggestions for strategies to safeguard your kidneys.

Chapter 3
Preventing Kidney Disease

Kidney disease is a dangerous illness that can affect people of all ages. However, it is often preventable. By making healthy living choices and getting regular checkups, you can help to protect your kidneys and keep them healthy.

How to Prevent Kidney Disease

There are a number of things that you can do to avoid kidney disease, including:

Control your blood pressure: High blood pressure is the top risk factor for kidney disease. Keeping your blood pressure under control can help to protect your kidneys.

Manage your diabetes: If you have diabetes, work with your doctor to keep your blood sugar levels under control.

Make healthy lifestyle choices: There are a number of other lifestyle choices that you can make to help protect your kidneys, such as:

Eating a healthy diet: A healthy meal is low in salt, potassium, and protein. It is also important to drink plenty of fluids, especially water.

Exercise regularly: Exercise helps to keep your blood pressure and blood sugar levels under control. It also helps to keep your weight down, which is important for kidney health.

Quit smoking: Smoking harms the kidneys and increases the risk of kidney disease.

Avoid dangerous substances: Avoid using illegal drugs and excessive amounts of drink. These chemicals can hurt the kidneys.

Eating a Healthy Diet

A healthy diet is one of the best ways to protect your kidneys. A healthy meal is low in salt, potassium, and protein. It is also important to drink plenty of fluids, especially water.

Sodium

Sodium is a chemical that can be found in many foods. Too much salt can raise your blood pressure, which can damage your kidneys. It is important to limit your intake of salt to 2,300 milligrams per day.

Potassium

Potassium is another chemical that can be found in many foods. Too much potassium can also be harmful to your kidneys. It is important to limit your amount of potassium to 4,700 milligrams per day.

Protein

Protein is an important food, but too much protein can be harmful to your kidneys. It is important to limit your intake of protein to 0.8 grams per kilogram of body weight per day.

Fluids

It is important to drink plenty of fluids, especially water. Water helps to flush out toxins from your body and keep your kidneys healthy. Aim to drink 8 glasses of water per day.

Exercise

Exercise is another important way to protect your kidneys. Exercise helps to keep your blood pressure and blood sugar levels under control. It also helps to keep your weight down, which is important for kidney health. Aim for at least 30 minutes of moderate-intensity exercise most days of the week.

Quit Smoking

Smoking harms the kidneys and increases the chance of kidney disease. If you smoke, quit as soon as possible. There are many tools available to help you stop smoking.

Avoid Harmful Substances

Avoid using illegal drugs and large amounts of drink. These chemicals can hurt the kidneys.

Getting Regular Checkups

It is important to get regular checkups, even if you do not have any signs of kidney disease. Your doctor can check your blood pressure, blood sugar, and kidney health. If you have any risk factors for kidney disease, your doctor may suggest extra tests.

Kidney disease is a dangerous illness, but it is often preventable. By making healthy living choices and getting regular checkups, you can help to protect your kidneys and keep them healthy.

Chapter 4

Managing Kidney Disease

Kidney disease is a serious issue that can affect your general health. If you have been identified with kidney disease, there are a number of things you can do to manage your health and improve your quality of life.

Treatment Options

The treatment for kidney disease will change based on the severity of your illness. In some cases, you may only need to make lifestyle changes, such as eating a healthy diet and moving regularly. In more serious cases, you may need to take medicine or even undergo dialysis or a kidney transplant.

Lifestyle Change

There are a number of living changes you can make to help control kidney disease. These include:

Controlling your blood pressure. High blood pressure is a big risk factor for kidney disease, so it is important to keep your blood pressure under control. Your doctor may recommend medicine to help you do this.

Managing your blood sugar levels. If you have diabetes, it is important to keep your blood sugar levels under control. This will help to protect your kidneys from further damage.

Eating a healthy meal. A good diet is important for everyone, but it is especially important for people with kidney disease. Your food should be low in salt, potassium, and phosphorus. You should also reduce your amount of protein.

Exercising regularly. Exercise can help to improve your general health and well-being, and it can also help to protect your kidneys. Aim for at least 30 minutes of moderate-intensity exercise most days of the week.

Medications

In some cases, you may need to take medicine to help control your kidney disease. These medicines may help to lower your blood pressure, control your blood sugar levels, or reduce the amount of protein in your pee.

Dialysis

If your kidneys are not working well enough to clean your blood, you may need to undergo dialysis. Dialysis is a process that takes waste products and extra fluids from your blood. There are two main types of dialysis: hemodialysis and peritoneal dialysis

Hemodialysis is a process that uses a machine to clean your blood. This is usually done three times a week for 3-4 hours each time.

Peritoneal dialysis is a process that uses your own body's cells to filter your blood. This is done by putting a catheter in your belly and filling it with a special fluid. The solution takes waste products and extra fluids from your blood, and then it is drained out of your body.

Kidney Transplant

A kidney transplant is a surgical process that replaces a sick kidney with a healthy kidney from a donor. This is the only cure for end-stage kidney disease.

Following Your Doctor's Instructions

It is important to follow your doctor's directions carefully if you have been identified with kidney disease. This will help to ensure that your situation is properly handled and that you receive the best possible care.

Managing kidney disease can be difficult, but it is important to know that you are not alone. There are many tools available to help you, including your doctor, a chef, and a kidney disease support group. With proper care, you can live a long and healthy life with kidney disease.

Additional Information

In addition to the information above, here are some extra things you should know about controlling kidney disease:

See your doctor regularly. It is important to see your doctor regularly so that they can check your health and make sure that your treatment plan is working.

Be aware of the signs and symptoms of kidney problems. These include swelling, tiredness, shortness of breath, nausea, vomiting, and changes in your pee.

Take care of your overall health. This includes eating a healthy diet, exercising daily, and controlling stress.

Get help. There are many tools available to help you deal with kidney disease, including support groups, online forums, and books.

Chapter 5
Living with Kidney Disease

Living with kidney disease can be challenging, but it is possible to live a full and active life. There are a number of things that you can do to manage your kidney disease and live well, including:

Taking care of your mental health: Living with kidney disease can be stressful. It is important to take care of your mental health by talking to a therapist or counselor if you need to.

Connecting with others: There are many support groups available for people with kidney disease. Connecting with others who understand what you are going through can be helpful.

Staying informed: There is a lot of information available about kidney disease. It is important to stay informed about your condition so that you can make informed decisions about your treatment.

Taking care of your body: Eating a healthy diet, exercising regularly, and getting enough sleep are all important for people with kidney disease.

Managing your stress: Stress can worsen kidney disease. It is important to find ways to manage your stress, such as yoga, meditation, or spending time in nature.

Taking Care of Your Mental Health

Living with kidney disease can be stressful. It is important to take care of your mental health by talking to a therapist or counselor if you need to. A therapist can help you to manage your stress, develop coping mechanisms, and improve your overall well-being.

Connecting with Others

There are many support groups available for people with kidney disease. Connecting with others who understand what you are going through can be helpful. Support groups can provide you with a sense of community, offer emotional support, and help you to learn more about your condition.

Staying Informed

There is a lot of information available about kidney disease. It is important to stay informed about your condition so that you can make informed decisions about your treatment. You can stay informed by reading books and articles about kidney disease, talking to your doctor, and attending support groups.

Taking Care of Your Body

Eating a healthy diet, exercising regularly, and getting enough sleep are all important for people with kidney disease. A healthy diet is low in sodium, potassium, and protein. It is also important to drink plenty of fluids, especially water. Exercise helps to keep your blood pressure and blood sugar levels under control. It also helps to keep your weight down, which is important for kidney health. Aim for at least 30 minutes of moderate-intensity exercise most days of the week. Getting enough sleep is also important for people with kidney disease. Sleep helps your body to heal and repair itself. Aim for 7-8 hours of sleep each night.

Managing Your Stress

Stress can worsen kidney disease. It is important to find ways to manage your stress, such as yoga, meditation, or spending time in nature. These activities can help you to relax and reduce your stress levels.

Living with kidney disease can be challenging, but it is possible to live a full and active life. By taking care of your mental health, connecting with others, staying informed, taking care of your body, and managing your stress, you can improve your quality of life and live well with kidney disease.

Chapter 6

The Latest Treatments for Kidney Disease

Symptoms of kidney disease

The signs of kidney disease can vary based on the severity of the illness. Early kidney disease may not cause any signs. However, as the disease continues, you may experience the following symptoms:

Fatigue

Trouble sleeping

Loss of appetite

Nausea

Vomiting

Weight loss

Muscle cramps

Foamy or red pee

Swelling in your hands, feet, or legs

If you experience any of these signs, it is important to see a doctor right away. Kidney disease can be a dangerous illness, but early diagnosis and treatment can help to avoid kidney failure.

Treatments for kidney disease

Hemodialysis

Hemodialysis is a process that takes waste products and extra fluid from the blood when the kidneys can no longer do it. It is usually done three times a week, for four hours each time. During hemodialysis, blood is taken from the body through a needle in the arm or leg. The blood then goes through a machine where it is filtered and cleaned. The cleaned blood is then returned to the body through another needle.

How does it work?

Hemodialysis works by using a machine to clean the blood. The machine has two parts: a dialyzer and a blood pump. The dialyzer is a big, hollow tube that is filled with a special filter. The blood pump moves the blood through the dialyzer.

The filter in the dialyzer takes waste products and extra liquids from the blood. The waste products are then cleared away, and the extra fluid is drained from the body.

Benefits of Hemodialysis

The perks of hemodialysis include:

It can be a life-saving medicine for people with kidney failure.

It can help to improve quality of life by clearing waste products and extra fluid from the blood.

It can also help to control blood pressure and blood sugar levels.

Risks of Hemodialysis

The dangers of hemodialysis include:

illness: Hemodialysis can increase the chance of illness.

Blood clots: Hemodialysis can increase the chance of blood clots.

Heart problems: Hemodialysis can increase the chance of heart problems.

Other complications: Other consequences of hemodialysis can include anemia, bone loss, and muscle cramps.

Peritoneal Dialysis

Peritoneal dialysis is a process that uses the lining of the belly to clean the blood. It is usually done at home, several times a day. During peritoneal dialysis, a special fluid is introduced into the belly through a catheter. The solution then flows in the belly for a period of time, filtering the blood. The fluid is then drained from the belly.

How does it work?

Peritoneal dialysis works by using the lining of the belly as a natural filter. The lining of the belly is called the peritoneum. The peritoneum is a thin, wet membrane that lines the inside of the belly.

During peritoneal dialysis, a special fluid is introduced into the belly through a catheter. The solution then flows in the belly for a period of time, filtering the blood. The fluid is then drained from the belly.

Benefits of Peritoneal Dialysis

The perks of peritoneal dialysis include:

It can be done at home, which gives people more freedom and ease.

It is less likely to cause blood clots than hemodialysis.

It may be better for people with heart troubles.

Risks of Peritoneal Dialysis

The dangers of peritoneal dialysis include:

illness: Peritoneal dialysis can increase the chance of illness.

Obstruction of the catheter: The catheter can become stopped or obstructed.

Hernia: A hernia can form at the place of the catheter insertion.

Choosing a Type of Dialysis

The best type of dialysis for a particular person will rely on their individual wants and preferences. Some things to consider include:

Lifestyle: Some people prefer hemodialysis because it is done in a center or hospital, while others prefer peritoneal dialysis because it can be done at home.

Health: Some people may not be able to handle hemodialysis due to health problems, such as heart disease.

Preference: Some people simply prefer one type of dialysis over the other.

Living with Dialysis

Living with dialysis can be difficult, but it is possible to live a full and busy life. People with dialysis need to be careful about their food and fluid intake, and they may need to take medicines to control their blood pressure and blood sugar levels. However, with careful planning and control, people with dialysis can live long and healthy lives.

Dialysis is a life-saving treatment for people with kidney failure. It can help to improve quality of life and increase life span. There are two main types of dialysis: hemodialysis and peritoneal dialysis. The best type of dialysis for a particular person will rely on their individual wants and preferences.

Chapter 7
Resources for Kidney Disease

There are many resources available to people with kidney disease. These resources can provide information, support, and practical help.

Information: There are many websites and organizations that provide information about kidney disease. These resources can help people to understand their condition, learn about treatment options, and connect with other people with kidney disease.

Support: There are also many support groups available for people with kidney disease. These groups can provide emotional support, practical advice, and a sense of community.

Practical help: There are also some organizations that provide practical help to people with kidney disease. These organizations can help people to find financial assistance, transportation, and home care.

Here are some of the resources available to people with kidney disease:

•	National Kidney Foundation: The National Kidney Foundation is a leading organization in the fight against kidney disease. The foundation provides information, support, and practical help to people with kidney disease.

•	United Network for Organ Sharing (UNOS): UNOS is the organization that manages the organ transplant waiting list in the United States. UNOS provides information about organ transplantation and helps people to find living or deceased kidney donors.

•	Kidney Disease Outcomes Quality Initiative (KDOQI): KDOQI is a program of the National Kidney Foundation that provides guidelines for the care of people with kidney disease. KDOQI's guidelines are used by doctors and other healthcare professionals to provide the best possible care for people with kidney disease.

•	Kidney Care Partners: Kidney Care Partners is a network of kidney care providers that offer comprehensive care for people with kidney disease. Kidney Care Partners' providers can help people to manage their condition, find a living or deceased kidney donor, and prepare for kidney transplantation.

How can I connect with other people with kidney disease?

There are many ways to connect with other people with kidney disease. Here are a few ideas:

•   Join a support group: There are many support groups available for people with kidney disease. These groups can provide emotional support, practical advice, and a sense of community.

•   Connect online: There are many online forums and chat rooms for people with kidney disease. These forums can provide a place to connect with other people who understand what you're going through.

•   Get involved with a patient advocacy organization: There are many patient advocacy organizations that provide support and resources

to people with kidney disease. These
organizations can also help you to connect with
other people with kidney disease.

Conclusion

Kidney disease is a serious condition, but it is not a death sentence. With early diagnosis and treatment, people with kidney disease can live long and healthy lives.

The information in this book has given you the power to take control of your kidney health. You now know the causes, symptoms, diagnosis, treatment, and prevention of kidney disease. You also know how to make healthy lifestyle changes to improve your kidney health.

I encourage you to use the information in this book to make positive changes in your life. By taking care of your kidneys, you are taking care of your overall health.

The Power of Knowledge

The best way to protect your kidneys is to be informed about kidney disease. This book has provided you with the knowledge you need to take steps to prevent kidney disease and manage your condition if you already have it.

The Power of Action

Now that you know what you need to do, it is time to take action. Make healthy changes to your lifestyle, and follow your doctor's instructions. With knowledge and action, you can take control of your kidney health and live a long and healthy life.

The Future of Kidney Health

The future of kidney disease is bright. There are many new treatments and technologies being developed that will improve the lives of people with kidney disease. There is hope that one day, kidney disease will be a thing of the past.

In the meantime, we can all do our part to help fight kidney disease. We can educate ourselves about the condition, we can support research, and we can donate to organizations that are working to find a cure.

Together, we can make a difference in the fight against kidney disease.

The Power of Hope

Hope is a powerful thing. It can help us to overcome challenges, it can give us strength, and it can help us to live our lives to the fullest.

If you are living with kidney disease, I encourage you to never give up hope. There is hope for a better future. With early diagnosis and treatment, you can live a long and healthy life.

I wish you all the best on your journey.